HERBAL REMEDIES FOR MIGRAINES

Unlocking Natural Relief With Herbs For Holistic Healing, Lasting Wellness, Vibrant Health And Healthy Lifestyle

DR. CARDEN KYRIE

DISCLAIMER

The only goal of this book is informational. Every effort has been taken by the author and publisher to ensure that the information provided is accurate. But the material in this book is given "as is," without any express or implied representation, warranty, or condition as to its accuracy, completeness, or suitability for any particular purpose.

Any loss, damage, or injury resulting from using the information in this book, or from any action or decision made as a result of such use, will not be covered by the author's or publisher's liability. It is recommended that readers seek the assistance of a certified specialist for guidance specific to their situation.

The opinions and viewpoints conveyed in this book belong to the author and may not necessarily represent the official stance or policies of any specified organizations or people. Any likeness to real-life occurrences, places, or people—living or deceased—is wholly coincidental.

No specific product, service, or therapy discussed in this book is endorsed by the author or publisher. Any reference to goods or services is made only for informative reasons and is not intended as a recommendation or endorsement.

Before making any judgments or acting on any information, readers are urged to independently confirm it all. Any unfavorable effects or repercussions arising from the usage of the material included in this book are disclaimed by the author and publisher.

By using this book, you consent to absolving the publisher and author of any and all claims, obligations, or losses resulting from your use of the material in it.

I appreciate your cooperation and understanding.

TABLE OF CONTENTS

CHAPTER ONE 8

  INTRODUCTION TO MIGRAINES 8

    SYNOPSIS OF MIGRAINES 8

    THE FUNCTION OF HERBAL TREATMENTS 9

CHAPTER TWO 12

  COMPREHENDING HEADACHE 12

    TYPES AND DEFINITIONS OF MIGRAINES 12

    REASONS AND INITIATORS 13

    SIGNS AND PROGNOSIS 14

CHAPTER THREE 16

  HERBAL REMEDIES AGAINST CONVENTIONAL TREATMENTS 16

    AN OVERVIEW OF TYPICAL TREATMENTS FOR MIGRAINES 16

    BENEFITS AND RESTRICTIONS 17

    COMBINING CONVENTIONAL METHODS WITH HERBAL 18

CHAPTER FOUR 20

  ESSENTIAL HERBAL COMPONENTS FOR RELIEVING MIGRAINES 20

    HISTORY AND TRADITIONAL USE 20

    SCIENTIFIC EVIDENCE AND STUDIES 20

    SUGGESTED DOSAGE AND PRECAUTIONS 21

    BUTTERBUR 22

    ADVANTAGES AND MODE OF ACTION 22

    POSSIBLE ADVERSE REACTIONS 23

    THE BEST USAGE PRACTICES 24

    GINGER 25

ADMINISTRATION AND PREPARATION 26

ANTI-INFLAMMATORY CHARACTERISTICS 26

BLENDING WITH ADDITIONAL HERBS 27

CHAPTER FIVE...30

HERBAL INFUSIONS AND TEAS 30

TEA WITH CHAMOMILE..30

EFFECTS OF CALMING THE NERVOUS SYSTEM.................30

TIPS FOR BREWING AND CONSUMING 31

TEA WITH PEPPERMINT...33

SELECTING PREMIUM PEPPERMINT LEAF 34

INFUSIONS OF LAVENDER 35

BENEFITS OF AROMATHERAPY FOR RELAXATION...........36

METHODS OF PREPARATION...36

CHAPTER SIX...38

LIFESTYLE AND DIETARY CONSIDERATIONS 38

IMPORTANCE OF HYDRATION...38

DIETARY TRIGGERS AND AVOIDANCE 39

STRESS MANAGEMENT TECHNIQUES 39

REGULAR EXERCISE AND ITS IMPACT.............................40

CHAPTER SEVEN 42

HERBAL REMEDIES FOR MIGRAINE PREVENTION 42

BUILDING A HOLISTIC PREVENTION PLAN......................42

COMBINING MULTIPLE HERBS FOR MAXIMUM EFFICACY.................43

MONITORING AND ADJUSTING THE HERBAL REGIMEN..................44

CHAPTER ONE

INTRODUCTION TO MIGRAINES
SYNOPSIS OF MIGRAINES

A common and crippling neurological condition, migraines have long baffled both medical professionals and the general public because of their complexity and range of symptoms. Those who experience these pulsating headaches frequently experience nausea, light and sound sensitivity, and a general decline in quality of life. Understanding the subtleties of migraines requires exploring the complicated interactions between hereditary, environmental, and lifestyle factors because migraines are a neurological disorder.

Recurrent, severe headaches that usually affect one side of the head and last anywhere from a few hours to several days are the hallmarks of migraines. Additional symptoms like visual abnormalities, aura, and cognitive impairment frequently accompany these episodes. Although the precise cause of migraines is still unknown, evidence points to a possible hereditary susceptibility combined with environmental triggers including stress, hormone fluctuations, and particular foods. A thorough approach to the prevention and therapy of migraines is necessary due to the complex web of factors that contribute to the condition.

THE FUNCTION OF HERBAL TREATMENTS

Herbal medicines have gained popularity in the field of migraine care as people look for non-conventional methods to lessen migraine attacks and relieve symptoms. For millennia, herbal remedies have been used in traditional medical systems throughout the world. These treatments are made from a variety of plant sources. Herbal therapies are popular because of their seeming natural source and generally have fewer negative effects when compared to traditional pharmaceutical treatments. However, it's important to approach the use of herbal remedies in migraine treatment with caution, taking into account both the potential advantages and disadvantages of each.

The complex interrelationship between nature and medicine is highlighted by the use of herbal treatments for migraines. Numerous herbs, including butterbur, ginger, and feverfew, have been studied for their ability to lessen the symptoms of migraines. For example, feverfew has long been used for its anti-inflammatory qualities and is thought to help lessen migraine frequency and intensity. Another herb that has shown promise in reducing migraines is butterbur. Clinical tests have shown this herb to be effective. Well-known for its anti-nausea qualities, ginger has also been studied for its possible function in reducing migraine-related symptoms.

Although using herbal medicines to treat migraines can be more gentle and comprehensive, it is important to practice caution when using them. Herbal therapies can vary greatly in their safety and efficacy, and it is important to carefully assess how they may interact with other drugs. Furthermore, it can be difficult to guarantee regular and dependable results because many herbal medications lack established dosages and formulas.

Comprehending migraines and investigating the possibility of using herbal remedies to treat them requires a careful analysis of the complex characteristics of this neurological condition. It is crucial to establish a balance between the rigorous examination of scientific investigation and the age-old wisdom of nature as we go deeper into the realm of traditional herbal therapy. This research could lead to a more thorough and individualized approach to treatment by giving people more resources to help them navigate the complex world of migraine management.

CHAPTER TWO

COMPREHENDING HEADACHE

TYPES AND DEFINITIONS OF MIGRAINES

Recurrent, intense headaches are the hallmark of migraines, a complicated neurological disorder that is frequently accompanied by other symptoms like light and sound sensitivity and nausea. These incapacitating headaches can impede a person's everyday activities for hours or even days. Since there are various kinds of migraines, each with unique characteristics, it's critical to comprehend the subtleties of this illness.

Migraine without aura and migraine with aura are the two main types of migraines. The majority of occurrences of migraine are of the more common kind, which is migraine without aura. It is typified by moderate to severe throbbing headaches, usually on one side of the head, with accompanying light and sound sensitivity and nausea. On the other hand, migraine with aura refers to particular neurological symptoms that either come on before or after the headache, such as tingling or blurred vision.

REASONS AND INITIATORS

Although the exact causes of migraines are unknown, a combination of environmental and genetic factors is thought to be involved. Given that those with a family history of migraines are more prone to get them, genetics is a major factor. Migraine onset is assumed to be related to changes in the brainstem and its interactions with the trigeminal nerve, a key pain channel. In addition, serotonin imbalances and other neurotransmitter abnormalities may contribute to migraine triggers.

The causes of migraines can differ from person to person and are varied. Some common causes are hormonal shifts in women, bright lights or strong aromas in the environment, and specific meals and beverages like chocolate, coffee, and aged cheeses. Part of managing migraines may involve recognizing and avoiding triggers.

SIGNS AND PROGNOSIS

Beyond merely headaches, migraines can cause other symptoms as well. Although they can affect both sides of the brain, migraines typically manifest as a throbbing or pulsating ache on one side. Sensitivity to light, sound, and odors are possible additional symptoms, along with nausea and vomiting. Aura symptoms might also appear in some people as tingling or numbness in the hands and feet, or as vision problems like flashing lights or zigzag lines.

A comprehensive medical history and physical examination are necessary for migraine diagnosis. Medical professionals should inquire about the frequency, kind, and accompanying symptoms of headaches as well as possible triggers. Imaging tests to rule out other underlying disorders, such as CT or MRI scans, may be ordered. Since there isn't a particular lab test for migraine diagnosis, the diagnosis is made based on the patient's reported symptoms and a clinical assessment.

Migraines are a complex neurological disorder with a variety of forms, intricate origins, and triggers. For efficient management and therapy, it is essential to comprehend the various facets of migraines, ranging from their definition and forms to their causes and triggers. People who have severe or chronic headaches should consult a doctor for a proper diagnosis and an individualized treatment plan.

CHAPTER THREE

HERBAL REMEDIES AGAINST CONVENTIONAL TREATMENTS

AN OVERVIEW OF TYPICAL TREATMENTS FOR MIGRAINES

Millions of people worldwide suffer from migraines, which are characterized by excruciating throbbing headaches that are frequently accompanied by nausea, light and sound sensitivity, and other health problems. Pharmaceutical medications, each intended to address a particular facet of the illness, are the standard treatment for migraines. NSAIDs, or nonsteroidal anti-inflammatory medicines, are frequently used to treat migraine-related pain and inflammation. Examples of these treatments include ibuprofen and naproxen sodium. Another class of medications called triptans relieves migraines by narrowing blood arteries and obstructing brain pain pathways. Furthermore, individuals who suffer from severe and regular migraines may be administered preventive drugs such as beta-blockers and anticonvulsants.

BENEFITS AND RESTRICTIONS

Traditional migraine therapies have benefits and drawbacks of their own. The quick and frequently dependable relief they provide for acute migraine episodes is one of their main advantages. For example, triptans can relieve pain quickly, which makes them especially useful for people who need relief from severe pain right away. However, these drugs have drawbacks as well, such as the possibility of unpleasant side effects like exhaustion, vertigo, and rebound headaches. Moreover, prolonged use of some drugs might result in tolerance and reliance, which eventually lowers their effectiveness. Furthermore, not every person responds well to traditional therapies, and others may have insufficient alleviation or negative side effects, which calls for the use of alternative methods.

COMBINING CONVENTIONAL METHODS WITH HERBAL REMEDIES

Growing interest has been seen in combining herbal medicines with conventional migraine medications in recent years to provide a more comprehensive approach to treating this illness. Some people believe that herbal treatments, which are frequently made from plants and other natural sources, are a more kinder option than prescription drugs. For instance, some people find that the anti-inflammatory herb feverfew helps to lessen the frequency and intensity of migraine attacks. Another herb that has shown promise in preventing migraines is butterbur; it lowers the frequency of attacks. It is important to remember, though, that although herbal medicines can seem to have a lot going for them, there is frequently no scientific proof of their effectiveness and their safety and potential combinations with prescription drugs need careful thought.

A more individualized and thorough approach to migraine therapy is made possible by the combination of herbal medicines and medical treatments. Some people may find comfort in combining prescription medications with herbal supplements, customizing their regimen to target certain symptoms and preferences. Combining these strategies calls for prudence though, as any potential interactions and contraindications need to be carefully considered. Those who are thinking about using herbal medicines should speak with medical professionals to be sure they can safely and successfully incorporate them into their current treatment plan.

Managing migraines requires a sophisticated knowledge of both traditional medical interventions and natural medicines. Although many people find quick relief from pharmaceutical medications, their drawbacks, and possible side effects encourage research into alternative therapies. Combining herbal medicines with conventional methods offers a more comprehensive approach to managing migraines, taking into account the various demands and reactions of each patient.

CHAPTER FOUR

ESSENTIAL HERBAL COMPONENTS FOR RELIEVING MIGRAINES

HISTORY AND TRADITIONAL USE

The scientific name for feverfew is Tanacetum parthenium, and it has a long and illustrious history in traditional medicine. Its use dates back to ancient Greece, where it was used for a variety of therapeutic purposes. Because the plant has historically been used to treat fevers, it has gained the popular name "feverfew." It was accepted as a treatment for headaches and migraines in addition to fever management. Feverfew has been an essential part of the herbal pharmacopeia for millennia since it was frequently employed by practitioners of traditional medicine to reduce inflammation and relieve pain.

SCIENTIFIC EVIDENCE AND STUDIES

Feverfew has been the subject of extensive scientific investigation in recent decades, particularly about its possible benefits for migraine relief. Its effectiveness in lessening migraine frequency and intensity has been investigated in several trials. Parthenolides, which are found in feverfew, are thought to be responsible for some of the plant's anti-inflammatory and vasodilatory properties. These characteristics might help lessen the vascular alterations brought on by migraines. Feverfew is still being researched in the field of complementary and alternative medicine for the treatment of migraines, despite conflicting results from various studies that indicate either conclusive or inconclusive evidence.

SUGGESTED DOSAGE AND PRECAUTIONS

Since there are differences in feverfew preparations and formulations, it is important to carefully examine the right dosage. It is frequently offered as tablets, capsules, or teas. Herbalists and medical professionals generally agree that you should begin with a low dose and raise it gradually as needed. Individual reactions can differ, though; therefore speaking with a medical expert is advised to determine the ideal dosage based on particular requirements.

Although feverfew has some potential advantages, it should be used with caution because it might cause allergic responses, gastrointestinal distress, and mouth ulcers.

BUTTERBUR

Petasites hybridus, the scientific name for butterbur, is a perennial shrub that is indigenous to Europe, portions of Asia, and North America. It has drawn notice due to its ability to treat migraines, a crippling illness marked by excruciating headaches frequently accompanied by nausea, light sensitivity, and visual abnormalities.

ADVANTAGES AND MODE OF ACTION

Butterbur's capacity to lessen headache frequency and intensity is one of its main advantages for migraine relief. Numerous studies have indicated the potential anti-inflammatory and vasodilatory effects of butterbur extracts, especially those that have been standardized to contain petasin and isopetasin. These processes are hypothesized to aid in the brain's blood arteries relaxing, which may lessen the vascular component linked to migraines.

Butterbur acts on multiple routes as part of its migraine-relieving mechanism. The active ingredients in butterbur, called petasins, are thought to prevent the body from producing inflammatory chemicals like prostaglandins and leukotrienes. Additionally, butterbur may interact with calcium channels to modify blood vessel tone, resulting in vasodilation. It is thought that this combined action on vascular control and inflammation is essential for treating the complex character of migraines.

POSSIBLE ADVERSE REACTIONS

Butterbur has some possible negative effects in addition to its potential advantages. The alkaloids pyrrolizidine found in raw or unprocessed butterbur can be harmful to the liver.

Consequently, to get rid of these dangerous substances, it is essential to use products that are readily available in the market and have undergone purification. Belching, indigestion, and minor allergic reactions are among the gastrointestinal problems that are frequently linked to Butterbur supplement side effects. Before adding Butterbur to a migraine treatment regimen, it is imperative to speak with a healthcare provider, particularly for those who already have liver issues.

THE BEST USAGE PRACTICES

It's critical to follow a planned treatment plan and adhere to suggested dosages when using Butterbur for migraine relief. For best results, standardized extracts with at least 15% petasins are frequently recommended. Furthermore, it is best to begin with a smaller dose and raise it gradually as tolerated. To guarantee safety and effectiveness, regular monitoring under the supervision of a healthcare professional is crucial. Moreover, people should take Butterbur in addition to their regular prescriptions unless directed otherwise by a healthcare provider. Butterbur should not be used as a stand-alone treatment.

Butterbur's anti-inflammatory and vasodilatory qualities make it a promising herbal ingredient for migraine relief. Comprehending the advantages, mode of operation, possible adverse reactions, and optimal applications is vital for those looking for a comprehensive method of migraine treatment. As with any herbal product, it's essential to speak with a healthcare professional to ensure a safe and customized integration into an all-encompassing migraine treatment regimen.

GINGER

Ginger's ability to relieve migraines has long been known, and its effectiveness can be linked to several important characteristics. A noteworthy feature is the strong anti-inflammatory qualities of ginger. Ginger contains anti-inflammatory properties that can help reduce the inflammation of blood vessels in the brain, which is frequently linked to migraines. Bioactive compounds found in ginger, like gingerol, have been researched for their potential to fight oxidative stress and reduce inflammation—two conditions linked to migraine symptoms.

ADMINISTRATION AND PREPARATION

There are numerous ways to take advantage of ginger's benefits for migraine treatment in terms of preparation and administration. Making ginger tea is a popular technique that involves steeping fresh ginger slices in hot water. This makes it possible to extract the beneficial ingredients, which makes consuming ginger in this way both convenient and calming. As an alternative, ginger can be added to food or taken as a supplement. Due to its adaptability in a variety of forms, ginger can be consumed by people with varying dietary habits and tastes.

ANTI-INFLAMMATORY CHARACTERISTICS

It's intriguing to investigate how ginger and other herbs work together to improve migraine treatment. It is possible to enhance the effects of ginger by combining it with other plants that have complementary characteristics. For example, combining ginger with turmeric, another plant well known for its anti-inflammatory qualities, could result in a potent combination that effectively prevents migraines. For a more all-encompassing method of treating migraine symptoms, herbs having migraine-relieving properties, such as peppermint, feverfew, or butterbur, can be strategically mixed with ginger.

BLENDING WITH ADDITIONAL HERBS

Ginger may help reduce migraine symptoms; this is evident from its anti-inflammatory qualities. Since inflammation is frequently a contributing component in migraines, people may find relief from the excruciating pain and discomfort connected to these episodes by including ginger in their daily routine. People have alternatives for incorporating this herbal treatment into their migraine management techniques because of the versatility of ginger in terms of preparation methods and its potential synergy with other herbs. Before making any major dietary or supplemental changes, as with any herbal therapy, it's best to speak with a healthcare provider, especially if you have any pre-existing medical conditions or are taking medication.

CHAPTER FIVE

HERBAL INFUSIONS AND TEAS
TEA WITH CHAMOMILE

Dried chamomile flowers are used to make chamomile tea, which is well known for its mild flavor and calming effects. For generations, people have loved this renowned herbal infusion because of its calming and stress-relieving properties. The Asteraceae family includes the chamomile plant, which is distinguished by its petite, daisy-like flowers with a bright yellow center. German chamomile (Matricaria chamomilla) and Roman chamomile (Chamaemelum nobile) are the two varieties of chamomile that are most frequently used in tea.

EFFECTS OF CALMING THE NERVOUS SYSTEM

Many people recognize that chamomile tea has a relaxing impact on the nervous system. Compounds in the tea, like apigenin, have sedative and anxiolytic properties. By attaching itself to particular brain receptors, apigenin helps to quiet the nervous system and promote relaxation. Furthermore, chamomile tea is frequently suggested as a natural insomnia treatment, improving the quality of sleep and helping individuals who experience restlessness.

TIPS FOR BREWING AND CONSUMING

It's important to know the right ways to boil and drink chamomile tea to reap its full advantages. Steeping the dried flowers in hot water is the basic method for making chamomile tea. For each eight ounces of water, add one to two teaspoons of dried chamomile flowers to make a cup. The ideal water temperature is 200°F, or 93°C, and steeping takes five to ten minutes on average. Extended steeping periods yield a more robust flavor; however, it's crucial to avoid over brewing since this could result in an aftertaste of bitterness.

You can drink chamomile tea plain or flavored with a little honey and lemon. A common way for people to wind down and relax before bed is to drink chamomile tea. It is a caffeine-free substitute that may be used regularly without giving off the same stimulating vibes as regular teas. Additionally, chamomile tea offers diversity in its intake since it can be served either hot or cold.

Store chamomile tea in a cold, dark place away from moisture and direct sunlight for maximum freshness. This guarantees that the subtle taste and healing qualities will last. Additionally, experimenting with various chamomile tea combinations, including those with lavender or mint, can yield interesting flavor profiles and improved calming effects.

In particular, chamomile tea is a mildly potent herbal infusion that has remarkably relaxing effects on the neurological system. Its extensive usage and lengthy history highlight how important it is for fostering general well-being. Through the practice of steeping and infusing chamomile tea into daily routines, people can fully utilize this herbal treatment for peace and relaxation.

TEA WITH PEPPERMINT

For decades, people have enjoyed the refreshing taste and several health advantages of peppermint tea, which is made from the leaves of the Mentha piperita plant. The potential of peppermint tea to reduce headache symptoms is one of its most notable benefits. Because of its well-known ability to relax muscles, the menthol found in peppermint leaves can help relieve tension in the head and neck. For individuals looking for a natural and calming solution for minor headaches or migraines, a warm cup of peppermint tea might be helpful.

Beyond its ability to reduce headaches, one of the most important factors in maximizing the health benefits of peppermint tea is selecting high-quality peppermint leaves. When choosing peppermint leaves for tea, freshness is the most important factor to consider. Choosing organic peppermint leaves guarantees that the tea is devoid of dangerous chemicals and pesticides.

A pungent, minty scent is indicative of high-quality peppermint, and it can be used to gauge how fresh the leaves are.

The method used to gather and dry peppermint leaves affects the tea's overall quality. When leaves are at their most flavorful and potent, they should be collected. The unique flavor and medicinal qualities of peppermint tea are largely attributed to the essential oils that are preserved in the leaves when properly dried. The best techniques are air or sun drying because they keep the leaves whole and don't lose any volatile oils.

SELECTING PREMIUM PEPPERMINT LEAF

In addition, steeping time and water temperature are important considerations while making peppermint tea. Water that is too cold might not extract the entire range of flavors from the leaves, while water that is too hot could produce a bitter taste. For steeping peppermint tea, a temperature of about 200°F (93°C) is ideal. To guarantee that the tea retains its pleasant and minty flavor without becoming too powerful, steep the leaves for around five to seven minutes.

In addition to its delicious flavor, peppermint tea has been shown to have possible health advantages, including the potential to reduce headache symptoms. To completely benefit from the medicinal qualities of peppermint tea, use premium leaves. Those who are mindful of freshness, harvesting practices, and brewing procedures can enjoy a cup of peppermint tea that is not only tasty but also a natural cure for a variety of illnesses.

INFUSIONS OF LAVENDER

Beyond the world of conventional teas, lavender infusions which are made from the fragrant lavender plant offer a wonderful and calming experience. Dried lavender flowers are steeped in boiling water to allow their essence to infuse the liquid with a pleasant and relaxing flavor. In addition to their distinct flavor, lavender infusions are prized for their numerous health advantages.

BENEFITS OF AROMATHERAPY FOR RELAXATION

One of the main advantages of lavender infusions is their calming aromatherapy benefits. Lavender has long been recognized for its relaxing characteristics, and when steeped in hot water, it produces fragrant components that can have a favorable effect on one's mood and stress levels. The pleasant perfume of lavender has been associated with lowering anxiety and providing a sense of tranquility. Enjoying a cup of lavender infusion might thus serve as a natural cure for individuals seeking relaxation and stress reduction.

METHODS OF PREPARATION

The methods of preparation for lavender infusions are simple yet vital to accessing the entire spectrum of flavors and benefits. To construct a great cup, start by selecting high-quality dried lavender flowers. Approximately one to two teaspoons of dried lavender per cup of water is a general guideline.

Boil water to slightly below boiling point and pour it over the lavender blossoms, allowing them to steep for around 5-7 minutes. This steeping time can be adjusted based on personal preference, with longer steeping times intensifying the lavender flavor. Straining the infusion before consumption ensures a smooth and enjoyable drinking experience.

For those who appreciate a twist to the traditional lavender infusion, experimenting with complementary herbs or flavors can add depth to the brew. Adding a hint of mint or a slice of lemon can enhance the overall taste profile while maintaining the calming essence of lavender. It's important to note that while lavender infusions are generally safe for most people, those with allergies or sensitivities to certain plants should exercise caution and consult with a healthcare professional if needed.

Lavender infusions go beyond being a simple beverage; they embody a sensory experience that combines taste, aroma, and therapeutic benefits.

CHAPTER SIX

LIFESTYLE AND DIETARY CONSIDERATIONS
IMPORTANCE OF HYDRATION

Hydration plays a pivotal role in maintaining overall health and well-being. Adequate water intake is essential for various bodily functions, including digestion, nutrient absorption, and temperature regulation. Water is a fundamental component of cells, tissues, and organs, and its importance cannot be overstated.

Dehydration can lead to a range of issues such as fatigue, headaches, and impaired cognitive function. To maintain optimal health, individuals should strive to consume an adequate amount of water daily, recognizing that factors such as climate, physical activity, and individual health conditions may influence hydration needs.

DIETARY TRIGGERS AND AVOIDANCE

Dietary triggers and avoidance are critical considerations for those seeking to optimize their lifestyle. Many individuals are affected by specific foods that can trigger adverse reactions, such as allergies or intolerances. Identifying and avoiding these triggers can significantly improve overall well-being. Furthermore, adopting a balanced and nutritious diet is essential for sustained health. Incorporating a variety of fruits, vegetables, lean proteins, and whole grains can provide essential nutrients and support the optimal functioning of the body.

STRESS MANAGEMENT TECHNIQUES

Stress management techniques are indispensable in the modern world where individuals often face various stressors in their personal and professional lives. Chronic stress has been linked to numerous health issues, including cardiovascular problems and mental health disorders. Engaging in activities that promote relaxation, such as meditation, deep breathing exercises, or hobbies, can help mitigate the effects of stress. Developing a personalized stress management routine is crucial for maintaining emotional equilibrium and overall mental health.

REGULAR EXERCISE AND ITS IMPACT

Regular exercise is a cornerstone of a healthy lifestyle, with far-reaching benefits for both physical and mental well-being. Physical activity contributes to cardiovascular health, weight management, and the prevention of various chronic conditions.

Beyond the physical benefits, exercise also plays a crucial role in mental health by reducing stress and anxiety, improving mood, and enhancing cognitive function. Finding a form of exercise that is enjoyable and sustainable is key to incorporating it into one's routine, whether it's walking, jogging, swimming, or engaging in team sports.

Lifestyle and dietary considerations play a central role in maintaining and promoting overall health. Hydration, dietary choices, stress management, and regular exercise collectively contribute to a holistic approach to well-being. Recognizing the importance of these factors and incorporating them into daily life can pave the way for a healthier and more fulfilling lifestyle.

CHAPTER SEVEN

HERBAL REMEDIES FOR MIGRAINE PREVENTION

BUILDING A HOLISTIC PREVENTION PLAN

Creating a holistic prevention plan for migraine involves considering various factors that contribute to the onset of headaches. It goes beyond merely addressing the symptoms and aims to address the root causes of migraines. Lifestyle modifications play a crucial role in this approach. Adequate sleep, stress management, and a balanced diet are fundamental components of a holistic plan. In addition to these lifestyle changes, incorporating herbal remedies can provide a natural and complementary way to prevent migraines.

Herbs such as feverfew, butterbur, and peppermint have been traditionally used for migraine prevention due to their anti-inflammatory and vasodilatory properties. Integrating these herbs into a comprehensive plan allows for a multifaceted approach that targets different aspects of migraine triggers. Moreover, the holistic approach considers the individual's overall well-being, emphasizing the importance of mental and emotional health alongside physical factors.

COMBINING MULTIPLE HERBS FOR MAXIMUM EFFICACY

While individual herbs may offer migraine prevention benefits, combining multiple herbs can enhance their efficacy. Each herb may have unique properties that target specific aspects of migraine triggers. For instance, feverfew is known for its anti-inflammatory properties, butterbur for its vasodilatory effects, and peppermint for its muscle-relaxant qualities. By combining these herbs, a synergistic effect may be achieved, providing comprehensive protection against various migraine triggers.

The combination of herbs should be carefully chosen based on their compatibility and potential interactions. Consulting with a healthcare professional or herbalist is advisable to ensure a safe and effective blend. This approach not only maximizes the therapeutic benefits but also allows for a personalized and tailored solution, considering the individual variations in migraine triggers and responses to herbal remedies.

MONITORING AND ADJUSTING THE HERBAL REGIMEN

As with any preventive plan, monitoring and adjusting the herbal regimen are essential steps in ensuring its effectiveness. Migraine triggers and individual responses to herbal remedies can vary over time. Regular assessment of the herbal regimen allows for necessary adjustments to accommodate these changes. This involves paying attention to the frequency and intensity of migraines, as well as any potential side effects from the herbal supplements.

Maintaining open communication with healthcare providers is crucial during this process. Professionals can offer guidance on dosage adjustments, potential interactions with other medications, and alternative herbal options if needed. Additionally, keeping a detailed journal tracking migraine patterns, herbal intake, and any changes in lifestyle factors provides valuable information for both individuals and healthcare providers in refining the preventive plan.

Building a holistic prevention plan involves a comprehensive approach that considers lifestyle modifications and incorporates herbal remedies. Combining multiple herbs enhances their efficacy by targeting different aspects of migraine triggers. Regular monitoring and adjustment of the herbal regimen ensure that the preventive plan remains effective and tailored to individual needs. This integrative approach not only addresses the symptoms but also promotes overall well-being for individuals seeking natural alternatives for migraine prevention.

www.ingramcontent.com/pod-product-compliance
Lightning Source LLC
Chambersburg PA
CBHW060848260726
48661CB00002B/667